Urine Therapy

The Perfect Solution for Oral Health,
Youthful Look and Variety of Illnesses

By

Dr. Jolie Connor

This book is dedicated to my two lovely daughters Anna and Bella for their support and encouragement.

TABLE OF CONTENTS

Chapter 1: The History and Culture of Urine Therapy: From Ancient Times to Modern Day

Chapter 2: The Science Behind Urine Therapy: Understanding the Composition and Benefits of Urine

Chapter 3: The Top Benefits of Urine Therapy: How It Can Help Improve Your Health and Appearance

Chapter 4: The Different Ways to Use Urine Therapy: From Internal

Consumption to External Applications

Chapter 5: The Myths and Misconceptions Surrounding Urine Therapy: Separating Fact from Fiction

Chapter 6: Preparing for Urine Therapy: Tips on How to Collect and Store Urine for Optimal Use

Chapter 7: Safety and Side Effects of Urine Therapy: What You Need to Know Before Trying It

Chapter 8: Combining Urine Therapy with Other Holistic Practices: Enhancing the Benefits of Urine Therapy with Other Modalities

Chapter 9: Success Stories and Testimonials: Real-Life Accounts of People Who Have Benefited from Urine Therapy

Chapter 1

The History and Culture of Urine Therapy: From Ancient Times to Modern Day

Urine therapy, also known as urotherapy, has been used for thousands of years. Urine therapy was first documented in ancient India, where it was utilized as a therapeutic remedy for a number of diseases.

Urine therapy has also been documented in ancient Chinese scriptures as well as the works of

Greek and Roman physicians. In reality, Roman troops are known to have used pee to treat their wounds and avoid infections.

Urine therapy has been utilized for a variety of goals throughout history, including medical, cosmetic, and spiritual reasons. Urine was revered as a sacred substance in many cultures, endowed with particular traits and powers.

Urine therapy was known as amaroli in India and was considered a part of yoga. It was claimed that drinking one's own urine first thing in the morning helped purify the body and mind. Amaroli was also thought to contain a mystical component that helped people achieve enlightenment and transcendence.

Urine therapy was utilized to cure a number of conditions in China, including tuberculosis, asthma, and even cancer. Urine was thought to have significant healing qualities by Chinese physicians, who used it in conjunction with other medicinal herbs and treatments.

Urine therapy was utilized for cosmetic purposes in medieval Europe, particularly for the treatment of skin disorders such as acne and psoriasis. Urine was thought to have antibacterial characteristics and was also utilized as a natural skin bleaching and brightening agent.

Urine therapy acquired popularity in alternative medical circles during the twentieth century, particularly in India and China. Proponents of natural health and holistic living also supported the practice, believing that urine therapy may assist to purify the body and promote general wellness.

Urine therapy is being practiced today by a small but committed group of people who swear by its healing abilities and benefits. While the practice remains divisive, many individuals are interested in the possible advantages of this old custom.

Despite its lengthy history and widespread use, urine treatment remains a relatively unknown procedure throughout much of the Western world. This could be owing to the taboo and shame surrounding the usage of urine, which many people regard as unsanitary or repulsive.

However, as more individuals get interested in natural and alternative types of medicine, urine therapy and its potential benefits are gaining popularity. While the practice is not for everyone, it is a fascinating element of human history and culture.

Chapter 2

The Science Behind Urine Therapy: Understanding the Composition and Benefits of Urine

Urine is a complicated fluid discharged by the urinary system that is produced by the kidneys. It is mostly made up of water, but it also contains other chemicals like as urea, creatinine, and electrolytes.

Urea, in particular, is a fundamental component of urine and is responsible for its characteristic odor and flavor.

Urea is a waste product created by the liver during protein breakdown and discharged by the kidneys.

While urine is commonly thought of as a waste product that should be discarded, it actually includes a range of minerals and substances that are beneficial to the body. Vitamins, minerals, enzymes, hormones, and antibodies are examples of them.

One of the primary advantages of urine therapy is its ability to aid in the detoxification of the body. Urine contains chemicals that can aid in the removal of toxins and other harmful substances from the body, such as heavy metals and pollution.

Urine therapy may also contain anti-inflammatory qualities, which can aid in the reduction of edema and inflammation throughout the body. This can be especially beneficial for people who suffer from chronic pain or illnesses like arthritis.

Urine therapy is thought to assist support the immune system in addition to detoxifying and anti-inflammatory qualities. Urine contains antibodies that can aid in the battle against infections and other pathogens, as well as hormones that can aid in the regulation of the body's natural defenses.

Despite these possible benefits, urine treatment remains a contentious practice with little scientific evidence to back it up. Some health professionals warn that eating significant amounts of pee can be hazardous to the body, causing electrolyte imbalances and other health issues.

Many supporters of urine treatment, on the other hand, claim that when used in moderation and under the supervision of a healthcare expert, it can be a safe and effective technique to boost general health and well-being.

Urine treatment has been utilized for cosmetic goals in addition to its possible health benefits. Urine is thought to include enzymes and other substances that can help enhance skin and hair health and appearance.

Some people, for example, say that using urine as a natural facial wash or hair rinse can help minimize acne, wrinkles, and other indications of aging. While there is little scientific proof to back up these claims, many people swear by the skin and hair advantages of urine therapy.

Overall, while urine treatment may appear unusual or distasteful to some, it is a fascinating and sophisticated discipline that has been utilized for ages by societies all over the world. While more research is needed to fully grasp its possible advantages and risks, many people are nevertheless interested in learning more about this ancient ritual.

Chapter 3

The Top Benefits of Urine Therapy: How It Can Help Improve Your Health and Appearance

While some may find the thought of drinking or utilizing urine for health and aesthetic purposes repulsive, proponents of urine treatment think it can have a wide range of good impacts on the body and mind. Here are some of the most important advantages of urine therapy:

- **Detoxification:** Urine contains components that can aid in the removal of toxins and other harmful substances from the body, such as heavy metals and pollution. Urine therapy, when eaten or applied topically, can aid to flush out toxins and support general detoxification.

- Urine therapy is thought to contain anti-inflammatory qualities, which can assist to reduce swelling and inflammation throughout the body. This can be especially beneficial for people who suffer from chronic pain or illnesses like arthritis.

- Urine contains antibodies that can aid in the battle against infections and other pathogens, as well as hormones that can aid in the regulation of the body's natural defenses. Urine treatment can assist to avoid sickness and promote overall health and wellness by boosting the immune system.

- **Digestive health:** Some supporters of urine therapy claim it can enhance digestive health by balancing gut bacteria and aiding good digestion. Drinking urine is thought to deliver helpful bacteria and enzymes that aid in digestion and assist good bowel movements.

- Urine includes enzymes and other substances that can help enhance the health and look of your skin and hair. Urine, for example, is thought to contain urea, a natural exfoliator that can help remove dead skin cells and improve skin texture. It is also thought to contain vitamins and minerals that can aid in the promotion of healthy hair development and the prevention of hair loss.

- **Oral health:** It is claimed that swishing urine in the mouth helps combat bacteria and improves oral health. This is due to urine's antibacterial capabilities as well as its ability to improve general immune system function.

- **Mental health:** Some supporters of urine therapy believe that it can improve mental health by reducing anxiety and depression.

This could be owing to the potential mood-regulating effects of urine chemicals like tryptophan and serotonin.

- **Improved energy and vitality:** It is thought that urine therapy provides a natural energy boost and increases vitality. This is because the nutrients and substances present in urine, such as vitamins, minerals, and enzymes, can aid in total energy production in the body.

While further research is required, some studies have revealed that urine treatment may have potential cancer-fighting qualities. One study discovered that urokinase, a chemical present in urine, may assist to limit the growth and spread of some types of cancer cells.

While the benefits of urine therapy may appear enticing, it is critical to proceed with caution and under the supervision of a healthcare practitioner. Drinking excessive amounts of urine or using it incorrectly can result in electrolyte imbalances and other health issues, therefore it is critical to utilize urine therapy professionally and with caution.

In conclusion, while urine treatment may appear to be a contentious and uncommon technique, societies all over the world have used it for millennia for its possible health and beauty benefits. Individuals may make informed decisions about whether or not to pursue this old tradition if they grasp the top benefits of urine therapy.

Chapter 4

The Different Ways to Use Urine Therapy: From Internal Consumption to External Applications

pee treatment is the practice of using pee for health and cosmetic purposes. While the thought of ingesting or utilizing pee may be repulsive to some, there are numerous ways to include urine therapy into your daily routine.

Here are some of the most prevalent applications for urine therapy:

Consumption on the inside:

Drinking pee is one of the most prevalent ways to use urine therapy. pee treatment supporters think that drinking pee can help to enhance the immune system, aid in cleansing, and promote general health and wellness. To drink pee, simply take a fresh sample and consume it right away.

Enema: An enema is another approach to employ urine treatment internally. An enema is a procedure in which a solution is used to cleanse the colon and encourage bowel movements. Urine treatment supporters think that using urine in an enema might assist to flush out toxins and promote healthy digestion.

External Use Cases:

Topically applied urine therapy: Urine therapy can also be applied topically to the skin. Proponents think that urine includes enzymes and other substances that can help enhance skin health and appearance while also fighting germs and other diseases. Simply apply urine to the skin and leave it on for a few minutes before rinsing it off.

Urine can also be utilized in hair care to improve the health and appearance of the hair. Urine, according to proponents, includes vitamins and minerals that can stimulate healthy hair development, as well as enzymes that can assist eliminate buildup and improve scalp health. To use pee as a hair treatment, simply apply it to the hair and scalp and rinse it out after a few minutes.

Eye drops: Some pee treatment supporters claim that using urine as eye drops might assist enhance vision and treat specific eye problems. However, utilizing urine in the eyes should be done with caution because it can be unpleasant and potentially hazardous.

Oral care: It is claimed that swishing pee in the mouth helps combat bacteria and improves oral health. This is due to urine's antibacterial capabilities as well as its ability to improve general immune system function. Swish some pee in your mouth for a few minutes before spitting it out to utilize it for oral care.

Bathing: Urine therapy can also be utilized to boost overall skin health and relaxation in the bath. Simply add a couple cups of fresh urine to the bathwater and soak for 20-30 minutes to use urine in the bath.

Precautions:

While urine therapy has the potential to provide health advantages, it is critical to proceed with caution and contact with a healthcare practitioner before attempting any new therapies. It is also critical to avoid utilizing urine therapy if you have certain medical issues, such as renal disease or urinary tract infections.

It is also critical to collect and use urine in a safe and sanitary manner. Use fresh pee and store it in a clean container. Urine that has been resting for an extended amount of time should not be used since it may contain hazardous bacteria.

Finally, there are numerous applications for urine therapy, ranging from internal intake to external applications. While the concept of using urine for health and beauty advantages may appear unusual, supporters of urine therapy think it can have a wide range of good impacts on the body and mind. However, it is critical to proceed with caution and use urine therapy properly and under the supervision of a healthcare practitioner.

Chapter 5

The Myths and Misconceptions Surrounding Urine Therapy: Separating Fact from Fiction

Urine therapy has been practiced for centuries in various civilizations around the world. Despite its extensive history, however, there are numerous myths and misconceptions about urine therapy that can make it difficult for consumers to understand its potential benefits. The following are some of the most popular myths and misconceptions about urine therapy, as well as the facts that disprove them:

Myth #1: Urine is a toxic waste product consisting of hazardous compounds.

While urine contains waste items that are filtered out of the body, it also contains helpful substances including urea, creatinine, and minerals. Urine, in fact, has been utilized in medical treatments for centuries and is still used today to make drugs and diagnostic tests.

Myth #2: Urine therapy is only for extreme health lovers and practitioners of alternative medicine.

While urine treatment is more widely employed by persons interested in alternative medicine, mainstream healthcare experts are becoming more interested in its potential advantages. In fact, urine therapy is now being studied for its potential to cure a variety of medical ailments, including urinary tract infections and skin diseases.

Myth #3: Drinking pee is risky and can cause illness or infection.

While drinking fresh pee may appear unappealing to some, there is no evidence that it causes any substantial health hazards. Urine, in reality, is sterile when it exits the body and contains antibacterial characteristics that may aid in the battle against some types of infections.

Myth #4: Urine therapy may cure any ailment or medical condition.
While urine therapy may have certain health benefits, it should be noted that it is not a cure-all for all ailments or

medical conditions. It should never be used in place of medical treatment and should always be done under the supervision of a healthcare practitioner.

Myth #5: Urine therapy is a fad with no scientific proof to back it up.

While scientific research on the potential advantages of urine therapy is limited, there is a growing amount of anecdotal evidence that suggests it may have favorable impacts on specific health concerns. Furthermore, several of the chemicals detected in urine have been researched for potential health advantages and are already employed in medical therapies.

Myth #6: Urine therapy can only be used internally and cannot be utilized topically or in other ways.

While urine therapy is commonly connected with internal intake, it can also be utilized topically or in other ways, such as hair treatments or bath additives. Many of the possible benefits of urine therapy are thought to be derived from therapeutic chemicals found in urine, which can be absorbed by the body in a variety of ways.

Myth #7: Urine therapy is a rapid remedy for any health or beauty issue.

While urine therapy may have certain health benefits, it is not a quick remedy for all health and beauty issues. Urine therapy should be used responsibly and under the supervision of a healthcare expert, as part of a holistic approach to health and wellness.

To summarize, there are numerous myths and misconceptions about urine therapy that might make it difficult for people to comprehend its potential benefits. However, by separating fact from fantasy and pursuing urine therapy with an open mind and under the supervision of a healthcare expert, some of the potential advantages of this ancient practice may be realized.

Chapter 6

Preparing for Urine Therapy: Tips on How to Collect and Store Urine for Optimal Use

If you want to pursue pee therapy, one of the most crucial things to think about is how to collect and store urine for best results. Proper collection and storage can assist ensure that your urine is free of pollutants and safe to use. Here are some suggestions for collecting and storing urine for urine therapy:

Select the best time of day for collection.

The first step in collecting urine for therapy is determining the best time of day to do it. Urine should be collected in the morning since it is most concentrated and contains the highest levels of helpful chemicals.

Make use of a clean container.

When collecting urine, it is critical to utilize a clean, contaminant-free container. You can use a sterile container or clean and disinfect it before using it. Containers composed of materials that may react with the urine, such as plastic or metal, should be avoided.

Take mid-stream urine samples.

Begin peeing into the toilet or other receptacle before placing the collecting container under the stream to collect mid-stream urine. This can assist guarantee that the urine is devoid of pollutants that may have entered the stream at the beginning or end.

Store urine correctly.

It is critical to carefully store urine after collecting it in order to prevent contamination and maintain its beneficial characteristics. Keep urine in a clean container with a tight-fitting lid and in a cool, dark place. Refrigeration can help keep urine fresh and prevent bacteria from growing.

Use a urine separator if possible.
Consider utilizing a urine separator if you want to collect urine on a regular basis for therapy. A urine separator is a device that separates urine from other waste products like feces in order to ensure that the urine is free of pollutants. Urine separators are available for purchase online or in medical supply stores.

Consume plenty of water.

Drink plenty of water throughout the day to ensure that your urine is properly hydrated and includes helpful chemicals. Dehydration can result in concentrated urine, which may not be as useful for therapy.

Avoid collecting urine while sick.

If you are ill or have an infection, you should avoid collecting urine for therapy until you have fully recovered. Urine collected while unwell may contain hazardous compounds that can aggravate your condition.

Consult a medical professional.

It is important to contact a healthcare practitioner before beginning urine therapy to confirm that it is safe and appropriate for your specific needs. A healthcare practitioner may advise you on correct collection and storage practices, as well as the dangers and advantages of urine therapy.

Finally, collecting and storing urine for urine therapy necessitates meticulous sanitation and correct storage practices. You may guarantee that your urine therapy practice is safe, successful, and beneficial for your unique health needs by following these suggestions and talking with a healthcare practitioner.

Chapter 7

Safety and Side Effects of Urine Therapy: What You Need to Know Before Trying It

While urine therapy has been utilized for centuries in numerous cultures for its alleged health benefits, it is crucial to emphasize that this procedure is not without hazards and adverse effects. Before attempting urine therapy, it is critical to understand the potential risks and adverse effects. Here are some things you should be aware of:

Concerns about safety:
Contamination

Contamination is one of the most serious safety problems with urine treatment. Urine can include hazardous bacteria, viruses, and other pollutants that, if swallowed or applied to the skin, can cause illness or infection. To decrease the possibility of contamination, proper collection and storage practices are required.

Reactions to allergens

Some people are allergic to certain components of urine, such as urea or ammonia. Skin irritation, rashes, and other symptoms can result from allergic responses. If you have a history of allergies or sensitivities, you should proceed with caution when attempting urine therapy.

Interactions between medications

Certain drugs may interact with chemicals found in urine, causing unpleasant side effects or reducing the medication's effectiveness. Before attempting urine therapy, it is critical to contact with a healthcare provider, especially if you are taking medication.

Kidney failure

People with kidney illness may be more likely to experience negative side effects from urine treatment. This is because the kidneys are in charge of filtering waste and poisons from the body, and urine treatment may put more strain on the kidneys.

Adverse Reactions:

Vomiting and nausea

When ingesting urine or using it topically, some people may feel nausea and vomiting. This can be triggered by the odor or taste of urine, as well as the body's natural reaction to eating anything it considers as waste.

Irritation of the skin

When pee is applied to the skin, it might produce irritation or dermatitis, especially if the skin is sensitive or the urine is not properly diluted. It is critical to test a tiny area of skin before applying pee to a larger area, and to dilute urine as necessary with water or other chemicals.

Dehydration

Because urine includes significant levels of salt and other waste materials, using it as a source of hydration may result in dehydration. In addition to using urine therapy, it is critical to drink enough of water and other fluids.

Imbalances in electrolytes

Electrolytes, which are minerals that help regulate fluid balance in the body, are found in urine. The use of urine treatment may result in electrolyte imbalances, which can induce unpleasant side effects such as muscle cramps, lethargy, or irregular pulse.

To summarize, while urine therapy may offer potential health advantages, it is critical to be aware of the potential safety risks and adverse effects before attempting it. Proper collection and storage practices, as well as prudence and consultation with a healthcare practitioner, can help to reduce hazards and guarantee safe and effective urine treatment use.

Chapter 8

Combining Urine Therapy with Other Holistic Practices: Enhancing the Benefits of Urine Therapy with Other Modalities

Urine therapy is just one of many holistic methods that can be utilized to improve one's health and well-being. Combining urine therapy with additional modalities may allow you to maximize the benefits and get even better outcomes. Here are some complementary holistic techniques to urine therapy:

Meditation

Meditation is a technique for quieting the mind and focussing on the present moment. It has been demonstrated to relieve stress, improve mental clarity, and induce calm and relaxation. Combining meditation with urine therapy can help you stay focused and grounded while also improving your overall sense of well-being.

Yoga

Yoga is a physical and spiritual discipline that entails stretching, breathing exercises, and meditation. It has been demonstrated that it improves flexibility, strength, balance, and general physical health. Yoga combined with urine therapy might help you gain physical and mental strength and flexibility.

Acupuncture

Acupuncture is an ancient Chinese medical procedure in which small needles are inserted into particular spots on the body. It has been proved to help with pain relief, mood enhancement, and overall health and wellness. Acupuncture combined with urine therapy can assist to balance the body's energy and promote recovery.

Aromatherapy

Aromatherapy is the use of essential oils to promote physical and emotional wellbeing. Essential oils are produced from plants and can be used in a variety of ways, including inhalation, application topically, and air diffusion. Combining aromatherapy and urine therapy can aid in relaxation, mood improvement, and overall well-being.

Herbal medication

Herbal medicine is the use of plants and plant extracts to enhance health and treat illness. Herbs can be utilized in a variety of ways, including brewing teas, applying topically, and taking supplements. Combining herbal medicine and urine therapy can aid in healing and overall wellness.

Massage treatment

Massage therapy is the technique of massaging the soft tissues of the body in order to promote relaxation, relieve pain, and improve general physical health. Massage treatment combined with urine therapy can assist promote relaxation, reduce tension, and improve general well-being.

While combining urine therapy with other holistic techniques might be useful, it is critical to speak with a healthcare practitioner before attempting any new modality. Some practices may be inappropriate for some people, or they may interact with drugs or medical problems. You may be able to improve your health and wellness by working with a healthcare expert and combining urine therapy with other techniques.

Chapter 9

Success Stories and Testimonials: Real-Life Accounts of People Who Have Benefited from Urine Therapy

Urine therapy has been used to treat a wide range of illnesses for ages. While some may find the practice strange, many people have claimed major changes in their health and well-being after implementing urine therapy into their daily routine. Here are some real-life success stories and testimonials from people who have used urine treatment to help them.

Better Digestive Health

"I had been suffering from digestive problems for years, and nothing seemed to help." I tried a variety of diets and drugs, but nothing worked. Then I came across urine therapy and decided to give it a shot. My stomach difficulties were fully resolved within a few days of beginning the practice. I now feel better than ever and have more energy than I could have imagined." - Sarah, 35

Improved Skin Health

"I've always had acne-prone skin and tried every treatment under the sun to get rid of it." However, nothing seemed to work. My skin has never looked better since I began utilizing urine therapy as a topical treatment. My skin is now shining and vibrant, and the acne is gone. I never thought I'd be one of those people who swears by pee therapy, but I've changed my mind." - Michael (27),

Immune System Enhancement

"I used to get sick all the time, and it seemed like I was always fighting a cold or the flu." I then began adding urine therapy into my regular regimen and haven't been sick since. My immune system has never been stronger, and I now feel much more capable of fighting off illness." Samantha is 42 years old.

Better Mental Health

"I'd been suffering from depression and anxiety for years, and nothing seemed to be helping." Then I started using urine therapy, and my mental health improved significantly. "I feel much more calm and centered, and my overall sense of well-being has significantly improved." - John, 50

Better Eye Health

"I had been suffering from eye problems for years and had even considered surgery to correct the problem." But then I began utilizing urine therapy as an eye drop, and my vision has greatly improved. I no longer require glasses, and my eyes are better than ever." - Lisa, 29

While these success stories and testimonials do not represent everyone's experience with urine therapy, they do show the potential benefits that the practice can give. Urine therapy should be done in conjunction with other holistic practices and under the supervision of a healthcare practitioner. Urine treatment, on the other hand, can be a valuable tool in achieving optimal health and well-being for those who have found success with the practice.

Made in United States
North Haven, CT
23 June 2025